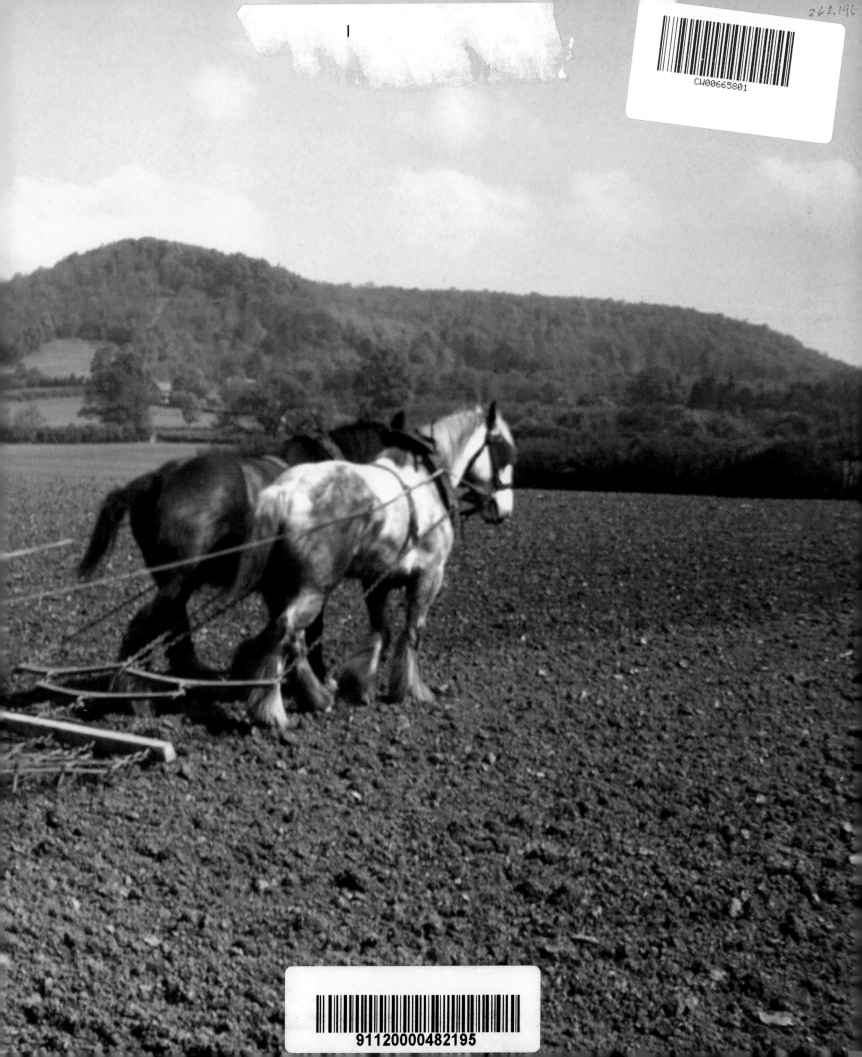

MEMORIES OF
WORKING LIFE
FROM THE
1950s & 1960s

Pictures
to share

Hard work beats talent,
when talent doesn't work hard.

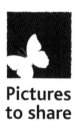

**Pictures
to share**

Published in 2019 by
Pictures to Share Community Interest Company,
a UK based social enterprise that publishes
illustrated books for older people.

www.picturestoshare.co.uk

ISBN 978-0-9934049-7-9

Front Cover:
Cobbler repairing shoes England, 1960s.
Contributor: Black Country Images / Alamy Stock Photo .

Front endpaper:
The English Scene. A field being ploughed by two horses, England, 1952.
Original Publication: Picture Post. The English Scene - unpub.
Photo by Raymond Kleboe / Picture Post / Hulton Archive / Getty Images.

Rear endpaper:
Rocking-horse workshop, Liverpool, October 1969.
Photo by SSPL / Getty Images. Credit: Manchester Daily Express.

Title page:
Working men talking outside their terraced homes in Britain, 1960s.
Contributor: Black Country Images / Alamy Stock Photo.

MEMORIES OF WORKING LIFE
FROM THE
1950s & 1960s

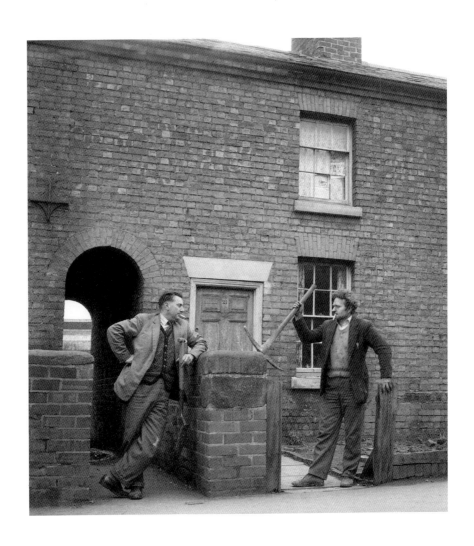

Edited by Michelle Forster

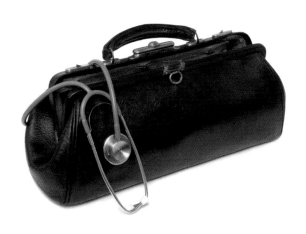

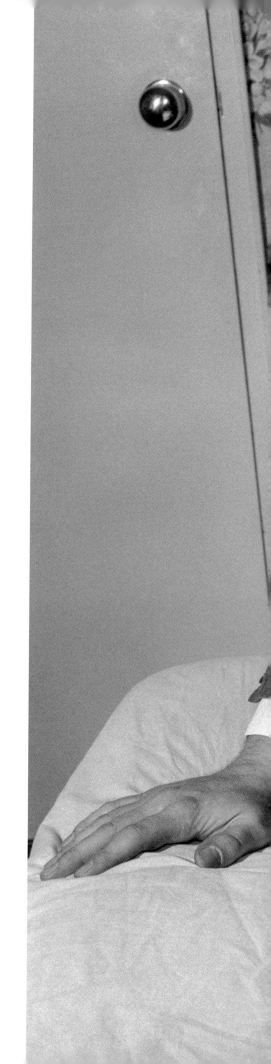

Doctors house calls were a regular occurrence in the 1950s and 1960s with over half of all of their appointments at patients' homes. A lot of people didn't have any transport to attend the Doctor's surgery so they made a lot of house visits and were supported by District Nurses.

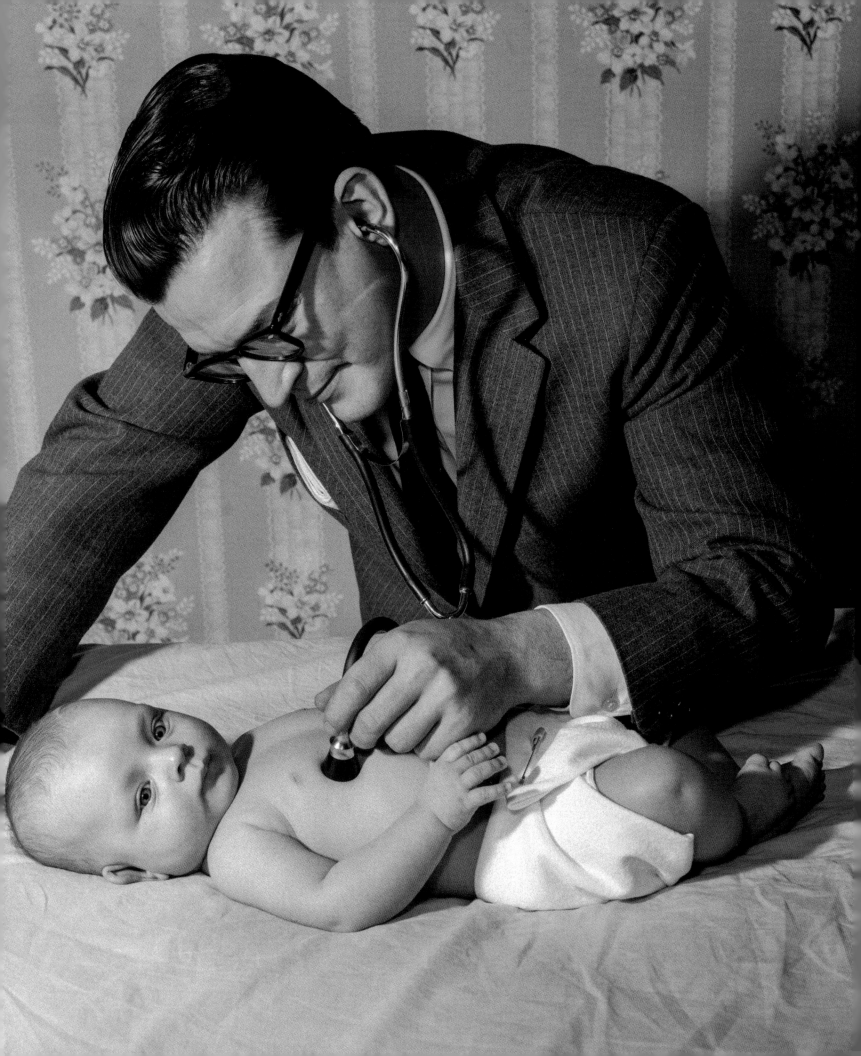

The **N**ational **H**ealth **S**ervice came into operation and District Nursing services become free for all patients for the first time in 1948.

By the end of 1958 there were 10,000 district nurses and midwives in England. They brought nursing care into every home, arriving on bicycles to help look after people of all ages. Often, they cycled 20 miles or more each day doing their rounds.

The District Nurse, out on her rounds visiting her elderly patients. Circa 1960.
Photo by WATFORD / Mirrorpix / Mirrorpix via Getty Images.

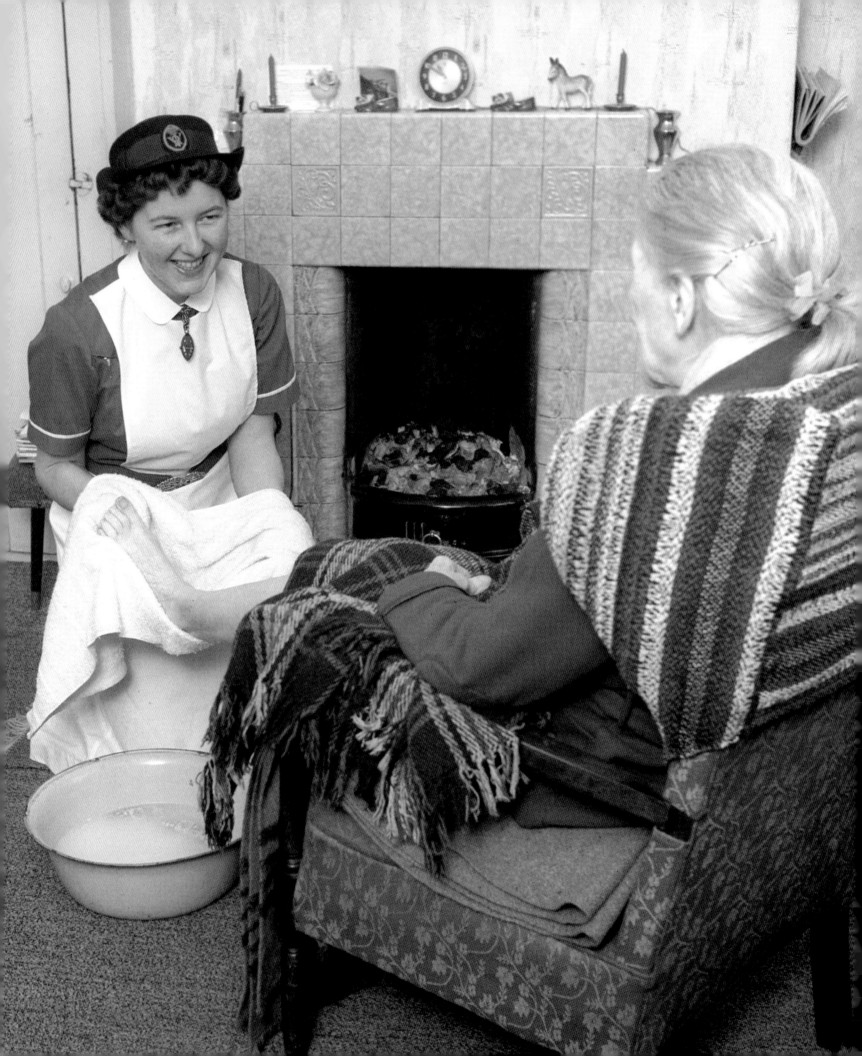

After the marriage ban was lifted in 1945 allowing married women to work, the increase in female teachers rose to around 70%, most of these taught in primary schools.

Male teachers were still in the majority at secondary and grammar schools.

A British lady teacher writing on a blackboard, 1955.
Contributor: Allan Cash Picture Library / Alamy Stock Photo.

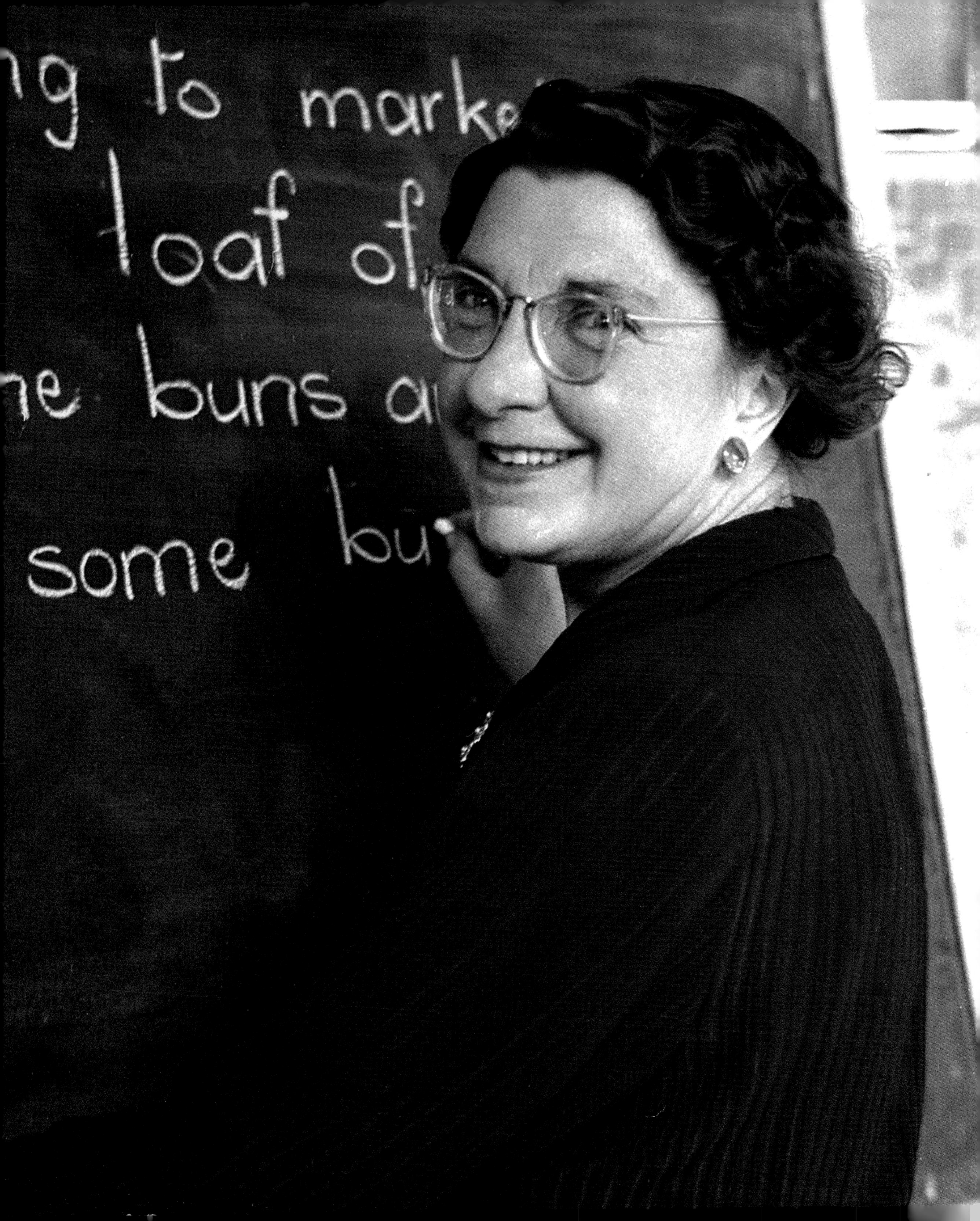
ng to marke
loaf of
ne buns a
some bu

A Woman's work is never done

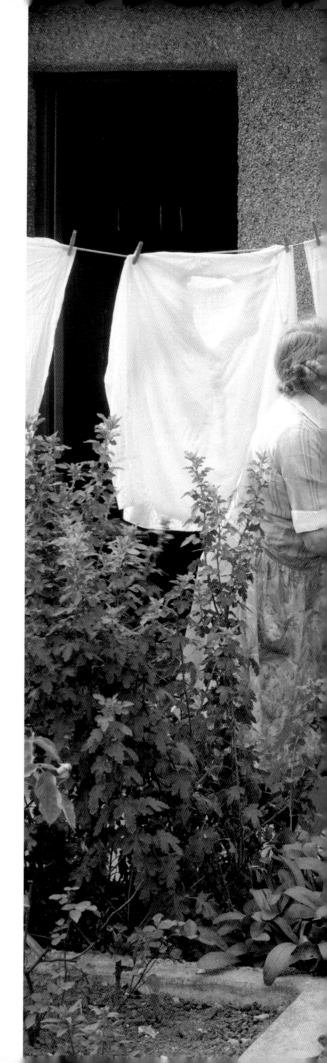

Woman hanging out the washing, 1955.
Contributor: Photo by SSPL / Getty Images.

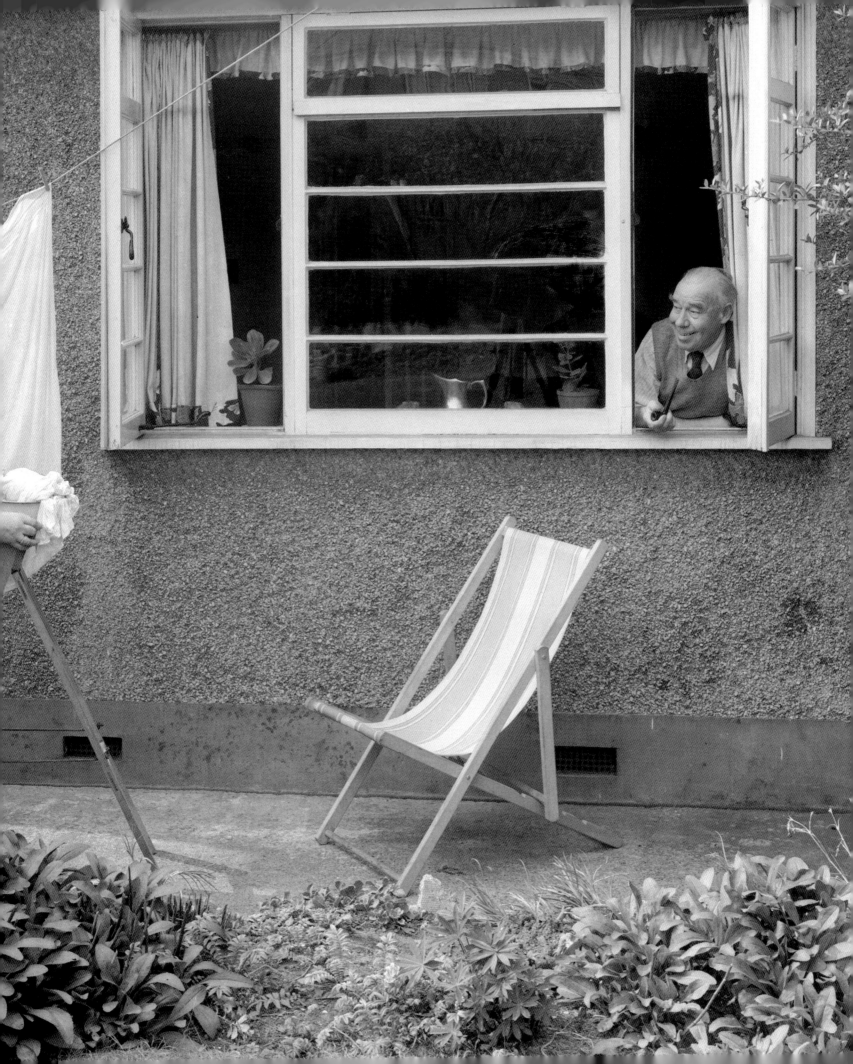

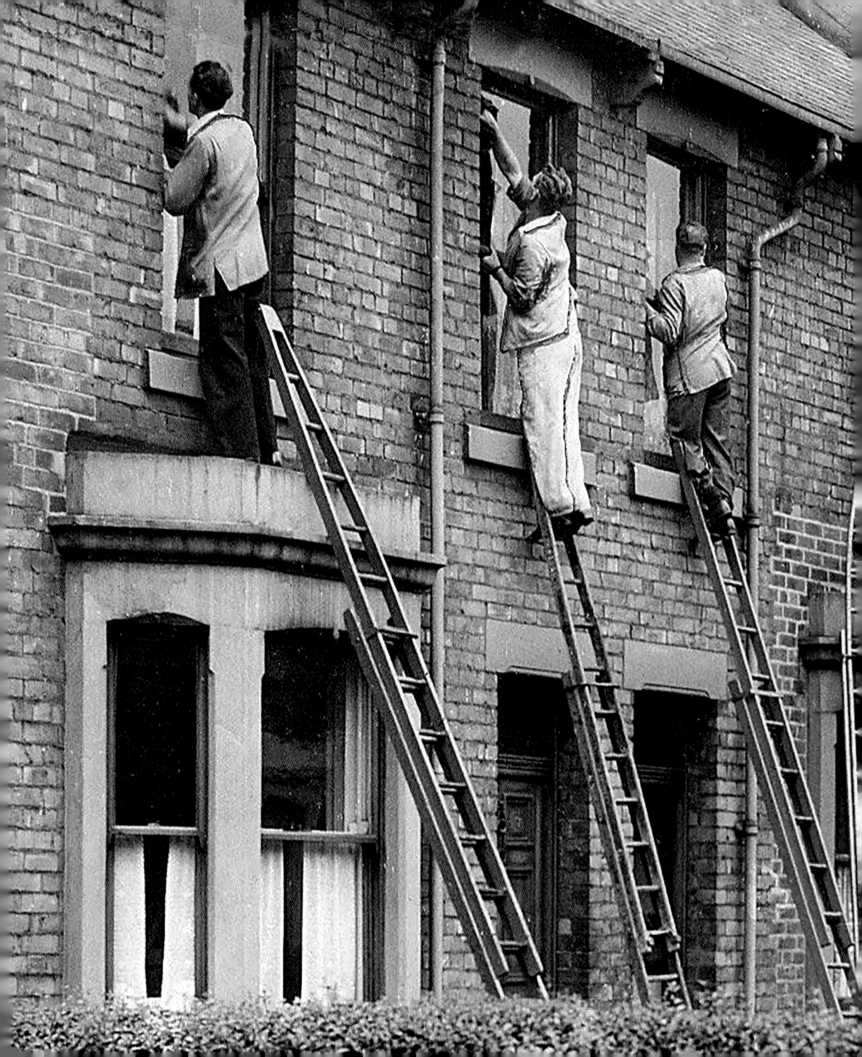

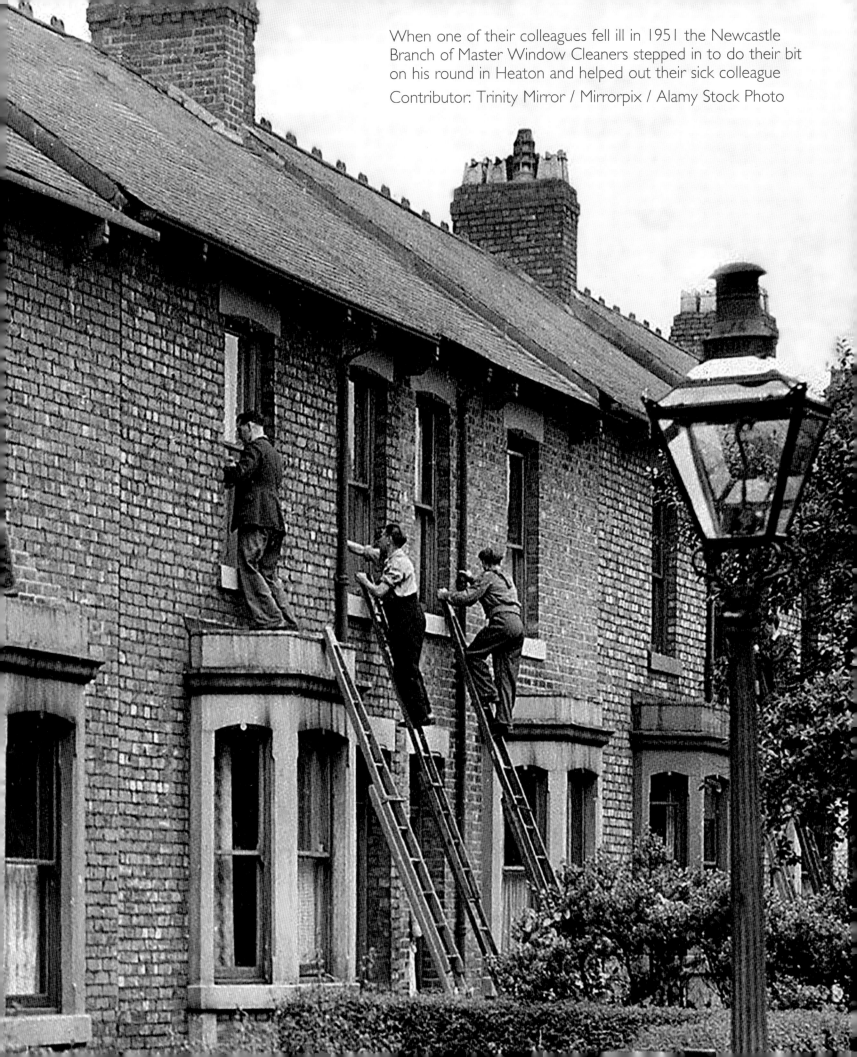

When one of their colleagues fell ill in 1951 the Newcastle Branch of Master Window Cleaners stepped in to do their bit on his round in Heaton and helped out their sick colleague
Contributor: Trinity Mirror / Mirrorpix / Alamy Stock Photo

No act of kindness, no matter how small, is ever wasted

Posting a Letter. A policeman helps a young child post a letter, 1950.
Photo by Keystone / Getty Images.

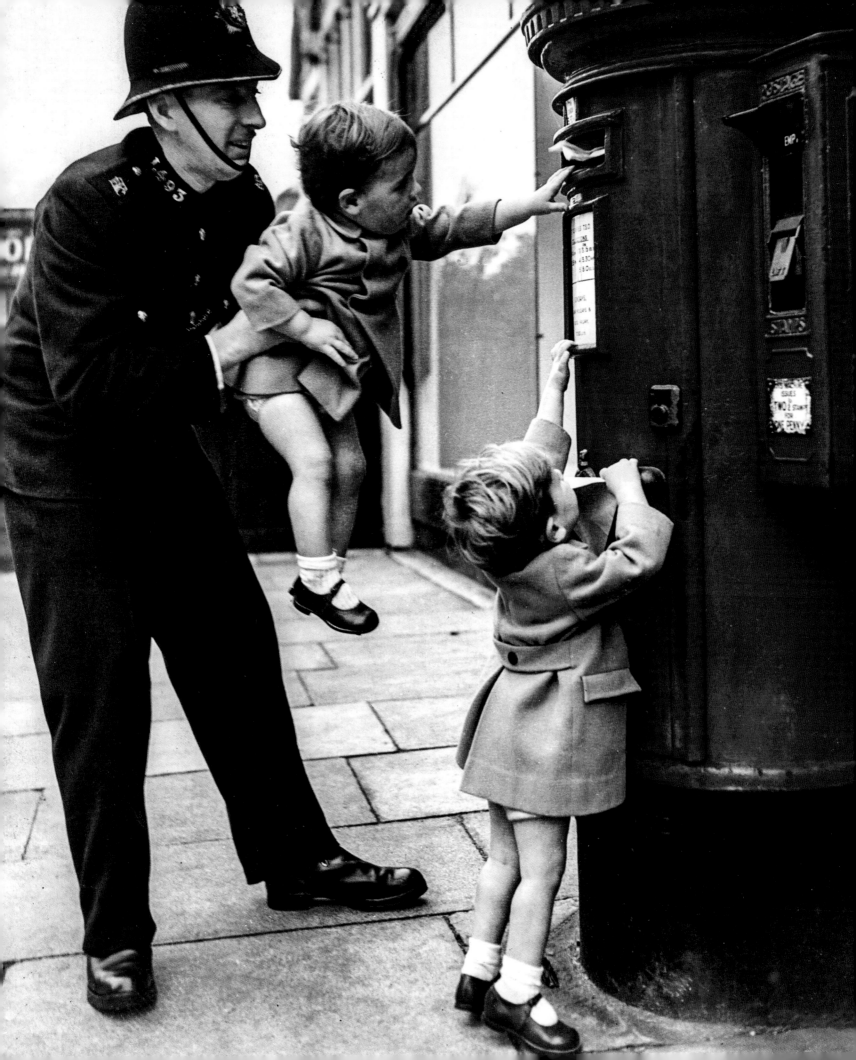

Some Mums went out to work for a few hours per day to be employed as a dinner lady at school.

Their main job was to prepare, cook and serve the food to the children. They didn't mind so much about table manners or finishing everything on the plate, they just wanted the children to go home having had a decent hot meal.

Popular pudding dishes served in the 1950s and 1960s were:

Rich Pudding
Semolina
Tapioca
Jam Roly Poly and Custard
Pink Custard

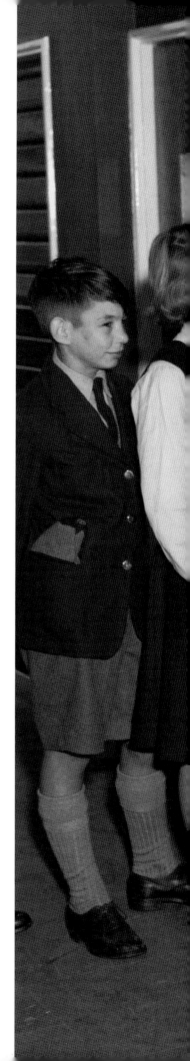

Children, Eltham Green Comprehensive in Woolwich, queue up to be served their school dinner.

Photo by © Hulton-Deutsch Collection / CORBIS / Corbis via Getty Images.

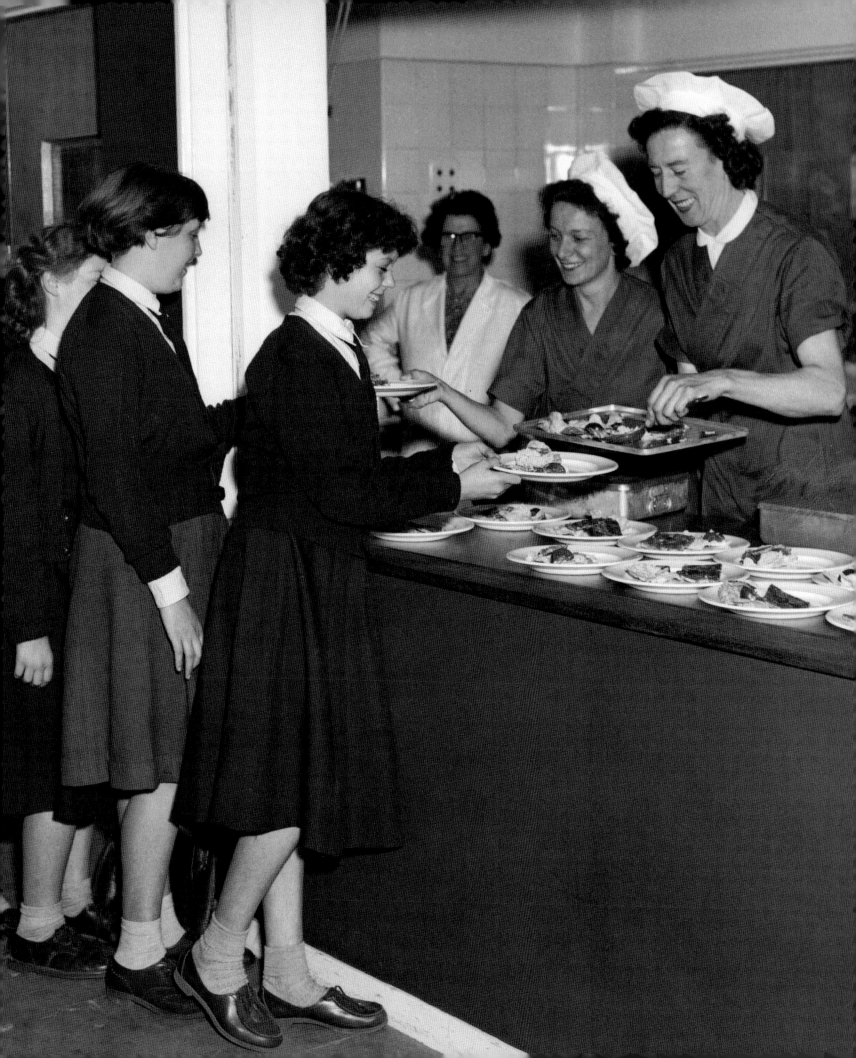

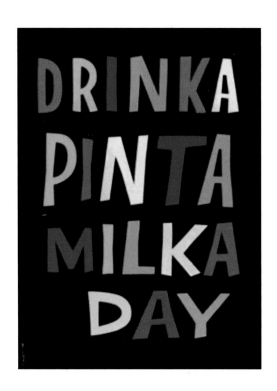

Milkmen would be up at 3am and would have finished their rounds soon after breakfast. Not only did Milkmen deliver milk they also delivered bread and potatoes. Around 99% of homes had their milk delivered daily. Not many houses had a fridge therefore daily deliveries were essential for homes to have fresh produce.

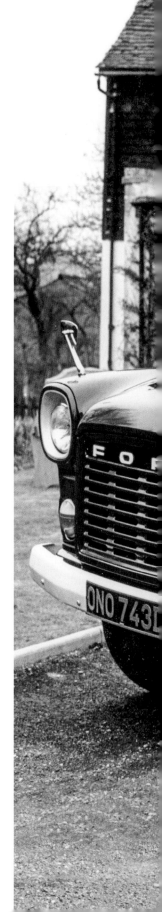

Ford milk float transit 1967.
Contributor: Motoring Picture Library / Alamy Stock Photo.

1959 poster on an advertising hoarding London -
it has the promotional slogan 'Drinka Pinta Milka Day'.
Contributor: M&N / Alamy Stock Photo.

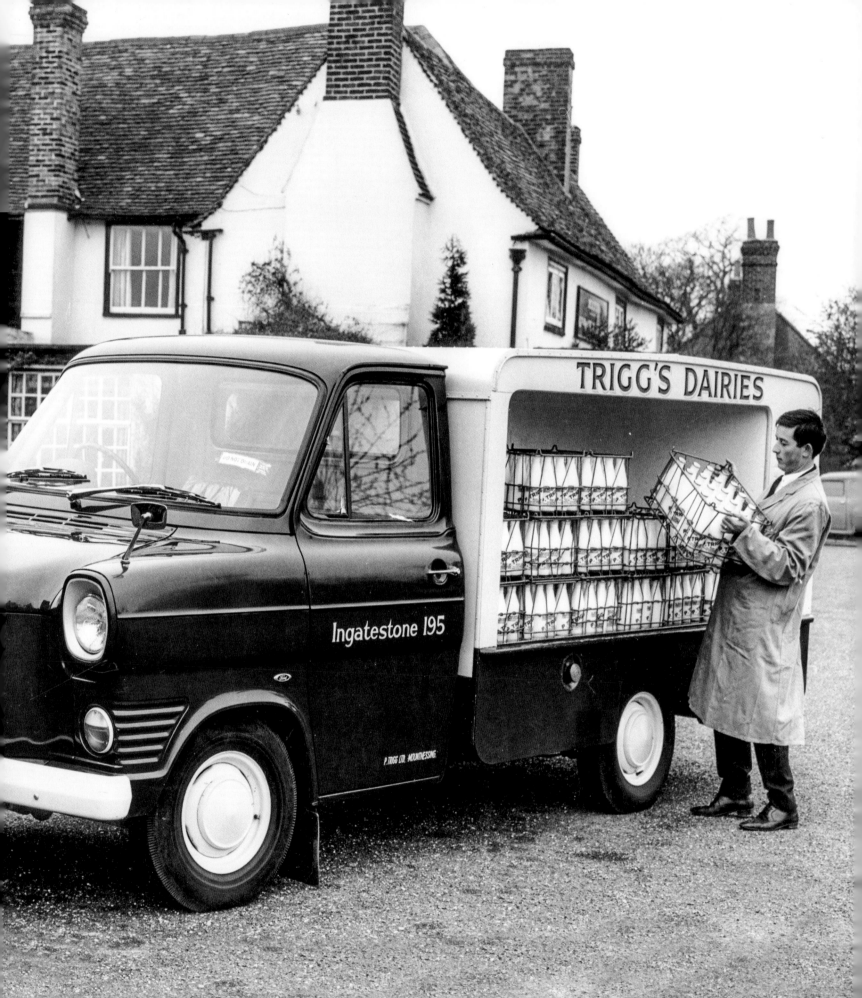

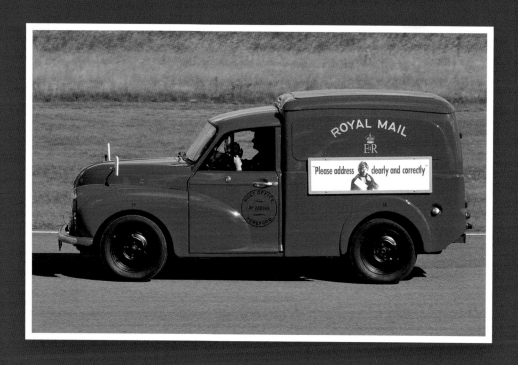

Due to the growth in mail volumes after the Second World War, it was realised that a nationwide post coding scheme was required to enable mail to be sorted automatically by machine. The first postcodes were introduced on a trial basis in Norwich in 1959 with the first three characters of the code ('NOR') representing the name of the city, and the last three characters of a particular street.

The task of coding the whole country was carried out in stages and was finally completed in 1974.

1964 Morris Mail Van.
Contributor: Shaun Finch - Coyote-Photography.co.uk / Alamy Stock Photo.

A postman pushing his bicycle up a hill in the village in Devon, 1954.
Photo by Carl Sutton / Picture Post / Hulton Archive / Getty Images.

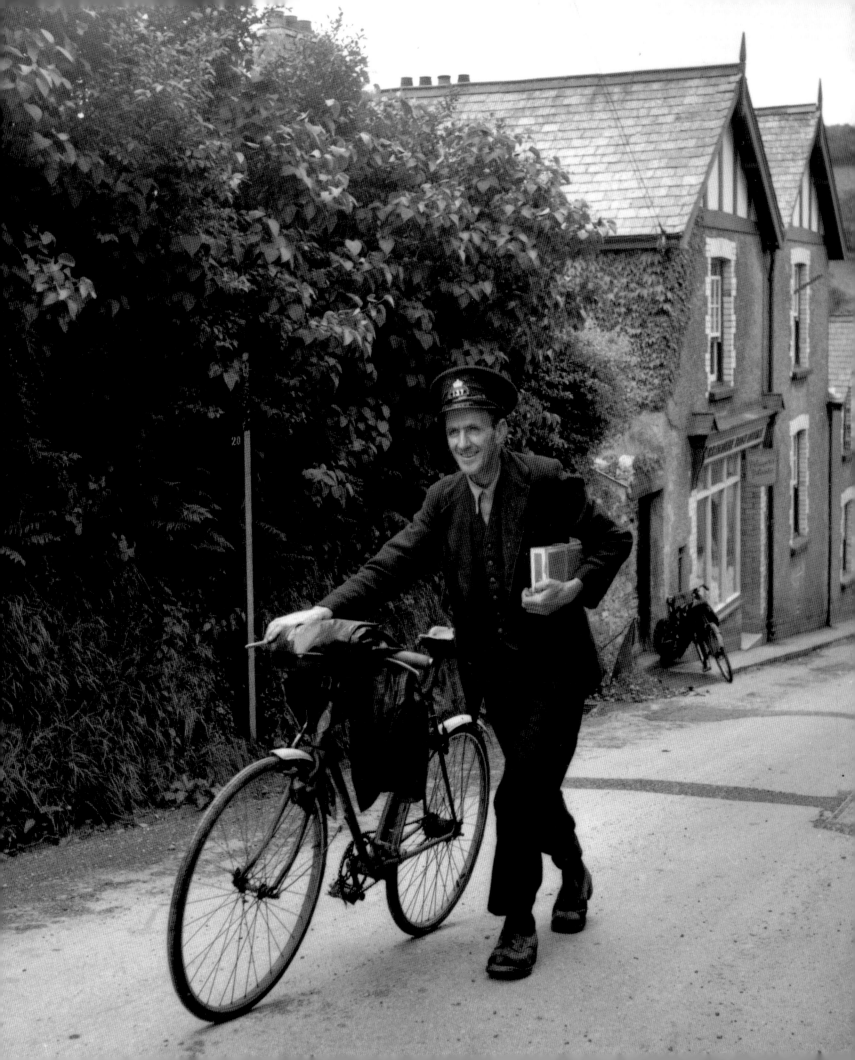

Apprenticeships were the most popular form of on-the-job training and there was a vast range of jobs and trades to choose from. School leavers at age 15 were encouraged to get qualified in a trade. Apprentices earned a small percentage of the full wage and had to wait around 5 years before they were qualified.

In the 1950s and 1960s some popular apprenticeships were:

Butcher	Hairdresser
Jockey	Electrician
Tailor	Secretary
Engineer	Mechanic

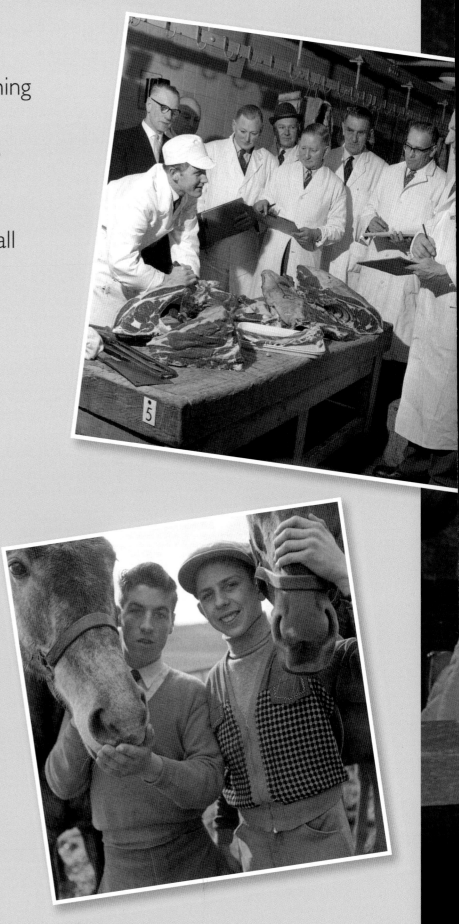

Apprentice jockeys with their mounts, UK, 1960. Photo by Daily Express / Getty Images.

Apprentice butcher showing his work to competition judges,1963, Meat Trades semi-finals. Photo by Paul Walters Worldwide Photography Ltd. / Heritage Images / Getty Images.

A Teenager has curlers put in her hair by a hairdresser stylist at a hair salon in London in 1962. Photo by Popperfoto / Getty Images.

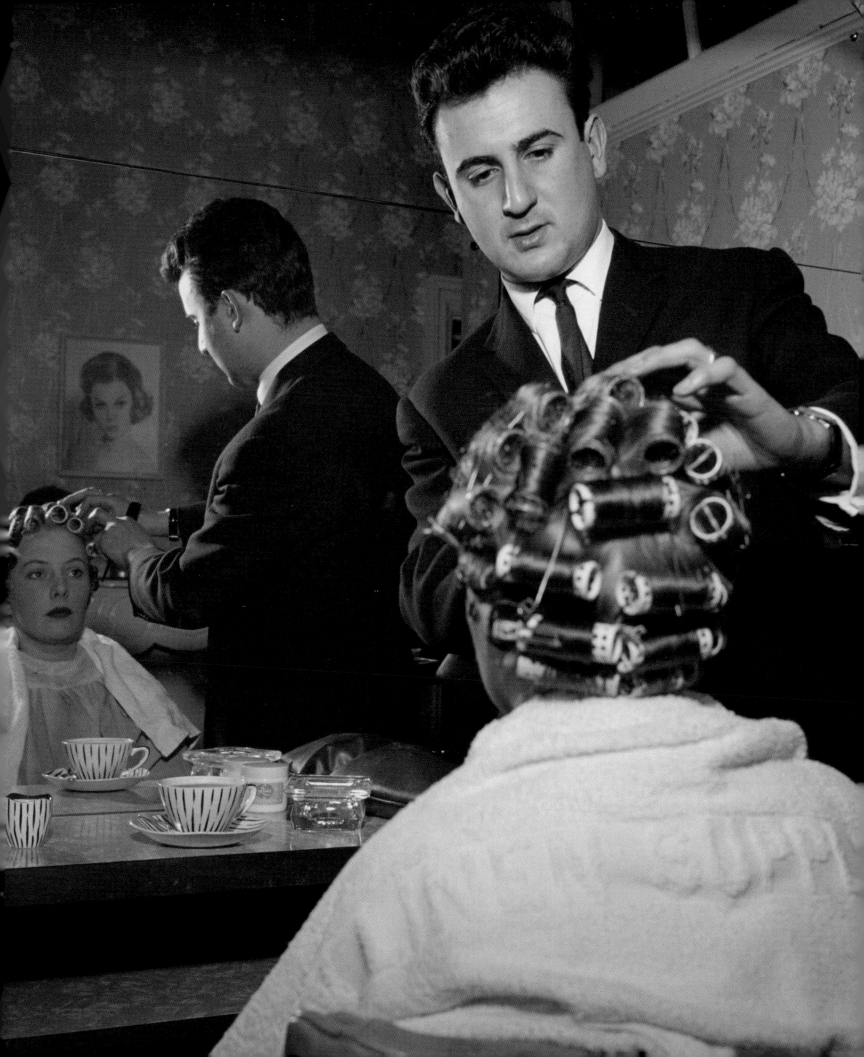

The Military

National Service slowed in the 1950s but continued right up until the early 1960s, there were four times as many servicemen in Britain back then as there are today.

In the early 1960s, a qualified RAF pilot earned about £1,200 a year. Today an RAF pilot is paid the equivalent of £1,900 in old money - earning about £40,000 a year.

World War II bomber pilots Group Captain Arthur Griffiths (left) and Squadron Leader Ken Hayward standing in front of a Lancaster Bomber at RAF Waddington, 1968.

Photo by Central Press / Hulton Archive / Getty Images.

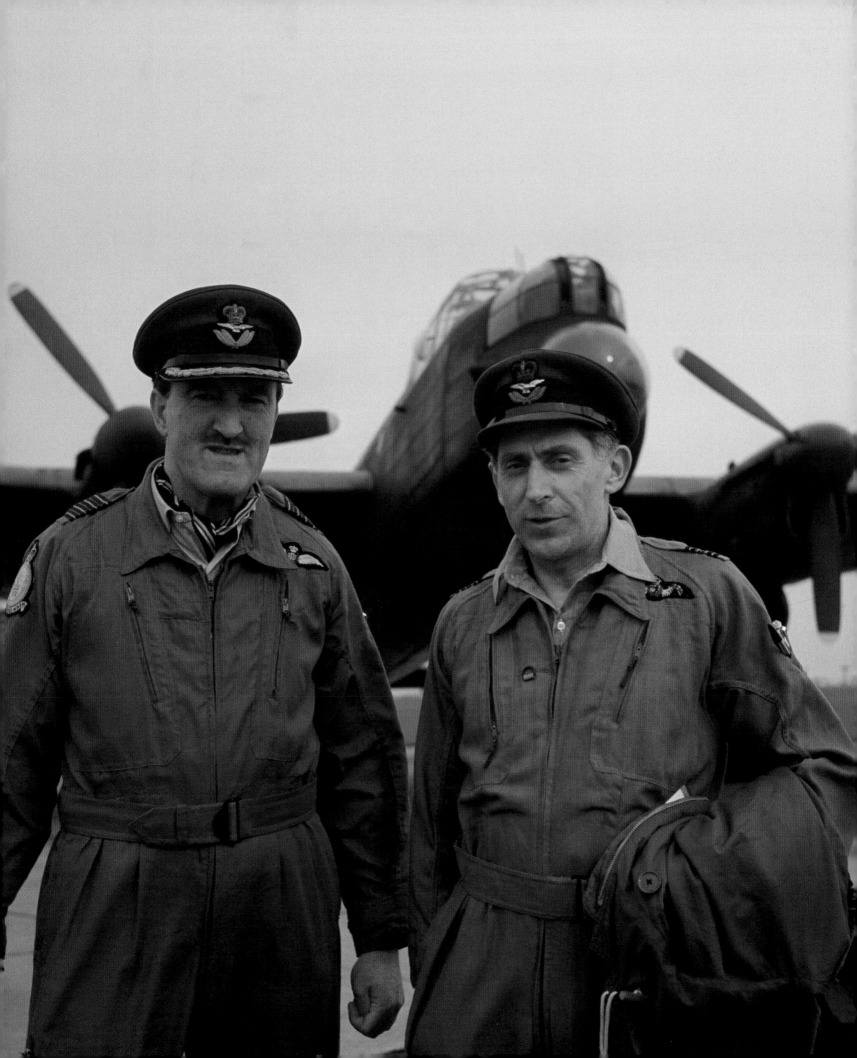

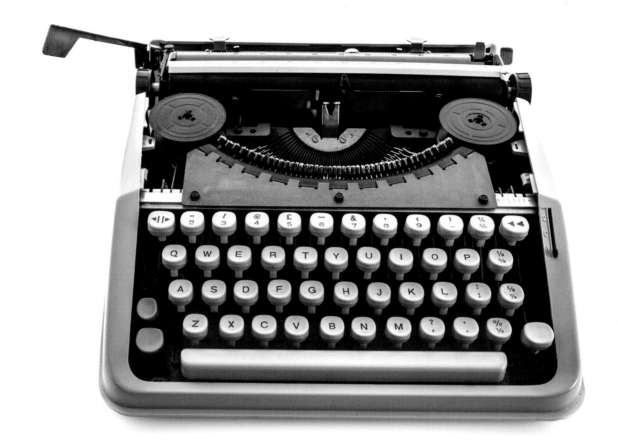

Training as a Shorthand Typist/Secretary

Training as a shorthand typist took a year after leaving school, usually at the local technical college, there were no shortage of jobs for shorthand typists.

Pitman Shorthand was the popular form of shorthand taught at college.

The typing was 'touch-typing' which meant that the typist was not to look at the keys while she typed. This was so that she could keep her eyes on her shorthand notebook.

Old Fashion Typewriter on a white background. Contributor: urbanbuzz / Alamy Stock Photo. Girls in typing class, late 1950s or early 1960s. Photo by Mark Jay Goebel / Getty Images.

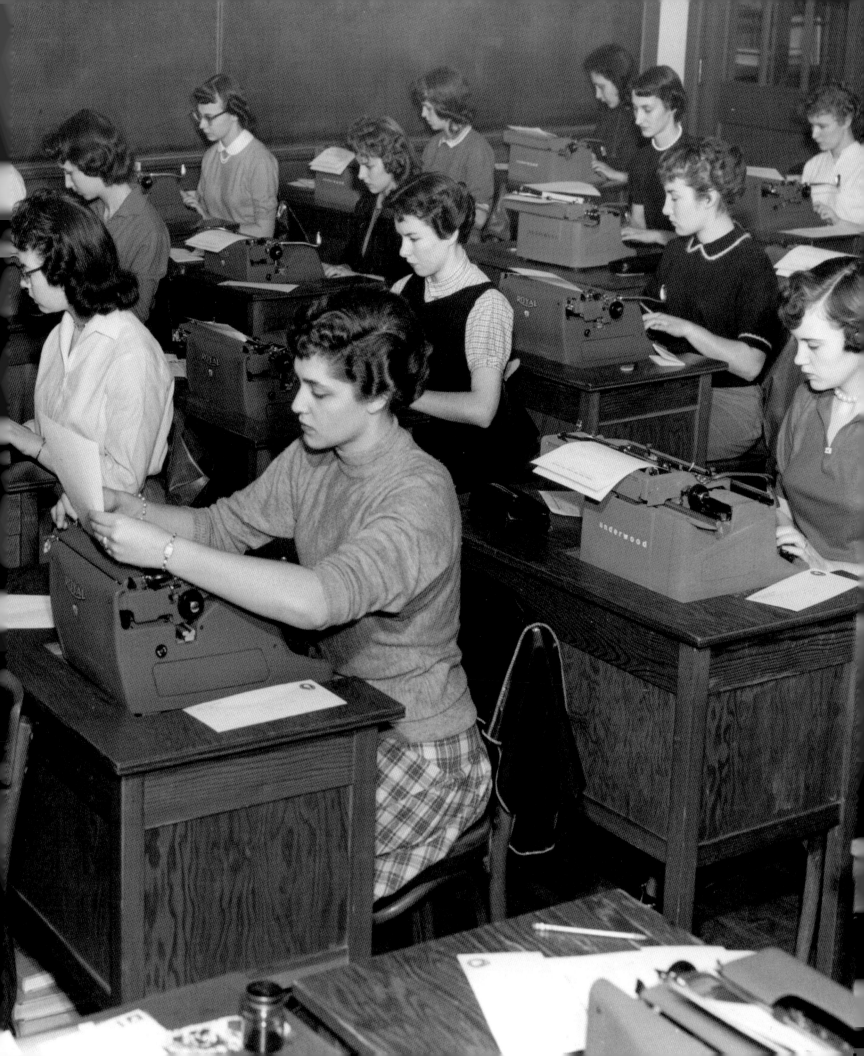

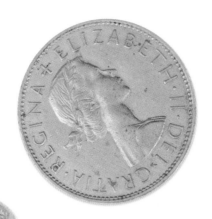

In the 1960s a typical sales assistant was paid £6 for a forty hour week, which is about 15p per hour.
Sales assistants, who joined at fifteen straight from school, were paid a junior rate of 7p per hour.

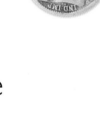

Full time workers worked five and a half days per week, including three Saturdays out of four. Shops employed Saturday Staff, who were normally still at school, and could be as young as thirteen. It was illegal for shops to trade on a Sunday.

Old English British silver pre-decimal coins, shillings, florins and three penny Contributor: Stephen Barnes / Finance / Alamy Stock Photo.

Staff stock up new Woolworth's Store, London Road, Liverpool, 14th November 1962. Photo by Liverpool Daily Post and Echo Archive / Mirrorpix / Getty Images.

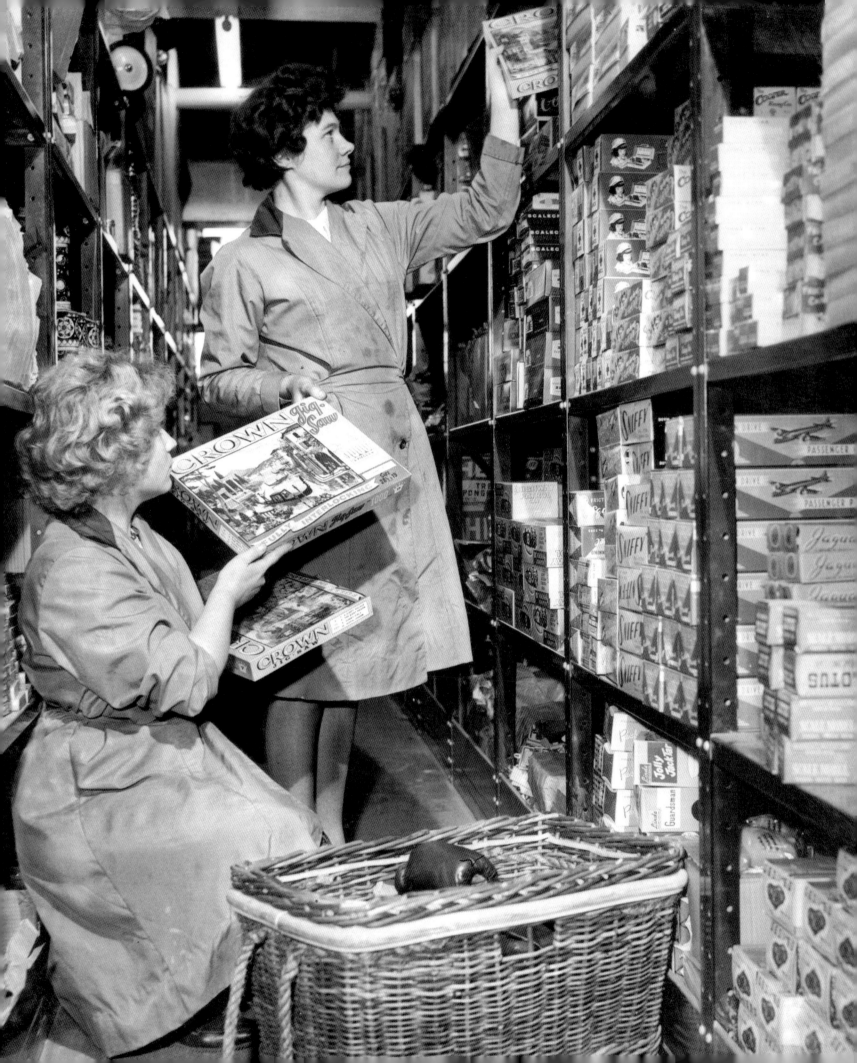

Housewife
& Mum

The 1950s and 1960s housewife took pleasure and pride in looking after her home and family. The role of the housewife was varied and included cooking, cleaning, shopping but most importantly nurturing her children and husband.

Most housewives had great friendship groups and could rely on each other for support, laughter and advice.

'The new Baby' is introduced to the neighbours, 1954.
Photo by George Greenwell, Daily Mirror / Mirrorpix / Getty Images.

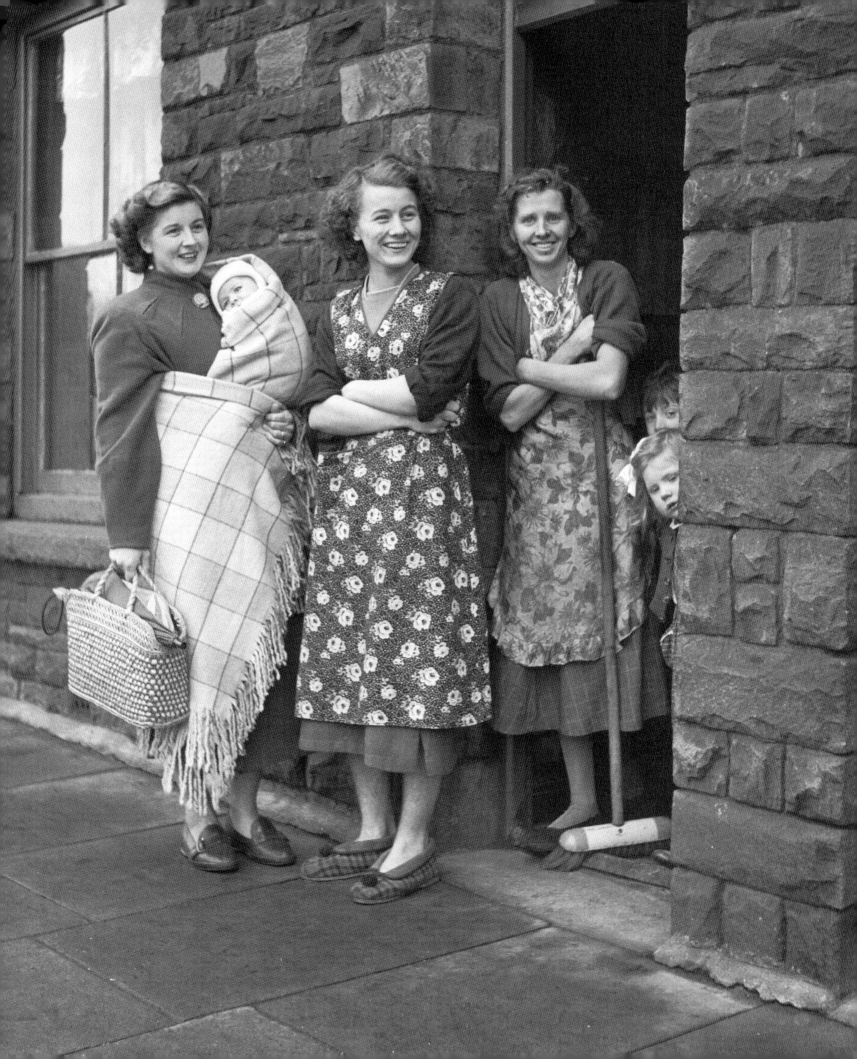

**Pictures
to share**

Graphic Design by Duncan Watts
Photo retouch by Studio 213

Published by
Pictures to Share
Community Interest Company.
Tattenhall, Cheshire
www.picturestoshare.co.uk

Printed in Europe through Beamreach Printing,
Cheshire, UK

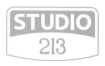
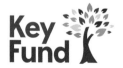

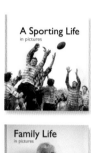
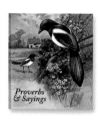
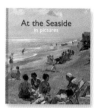
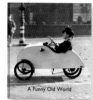
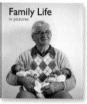
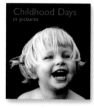
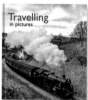

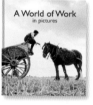

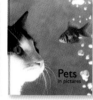

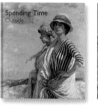

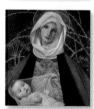
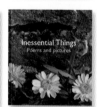
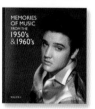
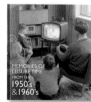
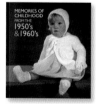
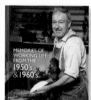

To see our other titles go to
www.picturestoshare.co.uk

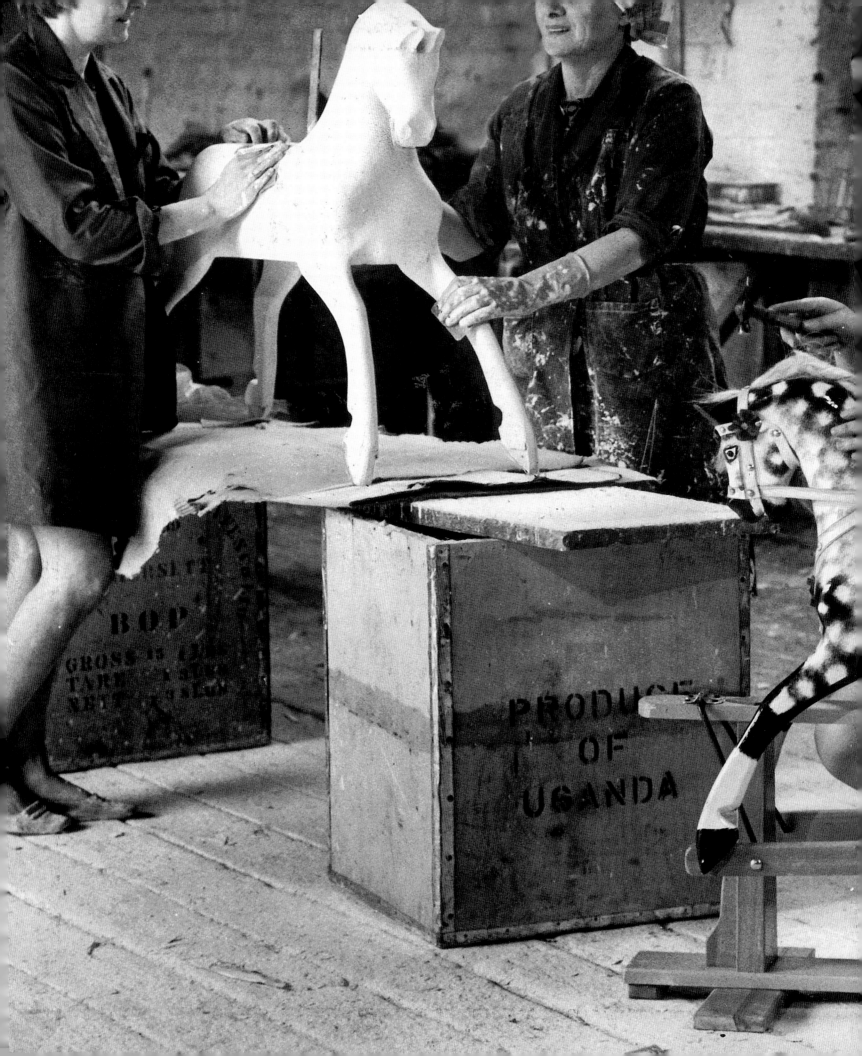